miracle juices™
health
remedies

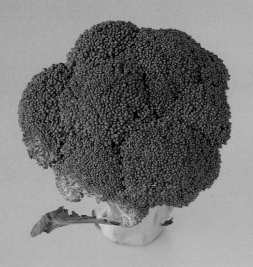

First published in Great Britain in 2002 by Hamlyn,
a division of Octopus Publishing Group Ltd
2–4 Heron Quays, London E14 4JP

Distributed in the United States and Canada by
Sterling Publishing Co., Inc.
387 Park Avenue South, New York, NY 10016-8810

ISBN 0 600 60696 1

A CIP catalogue record for this book is available
from the British Library

Printed and bound in China

10 9 8 7 6 5 4 3 2 1

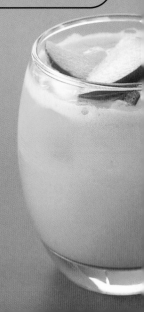

Contents

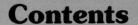

introduction

It would be a wonderful world if we were all fit and healthy, and free from disease, but unfortunately this just isn't the case. All too often our hectic lifestyles mean that we are stressed out, living and working in polluted environments, not exercising regularly and relying on stimulants such as tea, coffee, alcohol and cigarettes.

Even though we know we should be eating healthily and having at least five portions of fresh fruit and vegetables a day, the sad truth is very different. Many of us eat junk food and think sitting down to an evening meal means piercing the plastic film on a dish of processed food before popping it in the microwave.

It is no wonder that many people spend their time feeling tired and irritable, have trouble sleeping and always seem to be fighting off colds or other minor infections. This leads us to the doctor for painkillers and antibiotics, which may clear up the symptoms, but do not deal with the cause. In fact, regular courses of antibiotics upset the natural balance of our bodies by destroying not only the unwanted bacteria that are causing the infection, but also the beneficial bacteria in our digestive system as well. This can create another set of unpleasant symptoms. Read the list of possible side effects on any packet of prescribed drugs, they all tell the same story. It becomes a vicious circle, where our bodies are the ultimate losers.

Living like this over a prolonged period of time may weaken our immune systems to such an extent that it predisposes us to chronic degenerative diseases later in life.

By eating a balanced diet of fresh and, preferably, organic, food, we can strengthen our bodies and feel energized and healthy. If you are suffering from certain ailments, or determined to prevent further disease, there are many combinations of fruit and vegetables that can help if combined with a healthy eating plan that includes nutritious ingredients from the other vital food groups, such as proteins and fats.

So what makes fresh fruit and vegetables miracle remedies?

They are packed full of antioxidants, vitamins, minerals and enzymes that haven't been destroyed by processing and packing. Once fruits and vegetables have been juiced, the body assimilates their nutrients very rapidly. This can make them potent tonics. The juice is also a valuable source of water, which is essential to good health, particularly as many of the fluids we do drink deplete the body of vital water. Tea, coffee, alcohol, soft drinks and artificially flavoured drinks are all dehydrating to the system.

For those people who don't eat the recommended minimum five portions of fruit and vegetables a day, a juice will go a long way towards providing the body with those vital nutrients.

The juices in this book are aimed at certain conditions and will alleviate symptoms, and, if taken regularly, they will act as preventative agents in the fight against ill health. But they can't do it on their own.

In order to give yourself the best possible chance of remaining fit and full of vigour, you have to give it one hundred percent. Cut down on alcohol, junk food, tea, coffee and fizzy drinks, and give up cigarettes. Exercise regularly and eat nutritious food. Your body will love you for it.

common conditions

Condition	Juices that can help	Harmful influences
Anaemia	Iron Maiden, Heart Beet	Insecticides, excessive use of laxatives, tea and coffee (interfere with iron absorption)
Arthritis	Twister	Fatty foods, refined carbohydrates, excessive alcohol, food allergies
Bloating	Fine and Dandy, Bumpy Ride	Salty food, food allergies
Cellulite	Bumpy Ride, Fine and Dandy	Alcohol, smoking, junk food, lack of exercise
High cholesterol	Purple Passion, Heart Beet, Belly Berry	Saturated fats, stress, cigarettes, refined carbohydrates
Constipation	Way to Go, Healing Hand	Prolonged use of chemical laxatives, fatigue, stress, poor diet, lack of fluids
Diarrhoea	Belly Berry, Purple Passion	Bacterial infection from food poisoning, stress, antibiotics, dairy intolerance, alcohol
Eyesight	Twister, Vision Impeccable	Computers, fatigue, allergies, lack of A, C and E vitamins
Low fertility	Heart Beet, Earth Mother, Passion Thriller, Cool Down	Stress, poor diet, alcohol, smoking, caffeine

Condition	Juices that can help	Harmful influences
Heart disease	Heart Beet, Bumpy Ride, Purple Passion	Heavy meals, refined starches, hydrogenated and saturated fats, sugar
Menopause	Cool Down, Heart Beet	Refined food, alcohol
Motion sickness	Quantum Leap	Fatty foods, alcohol, stress, certain drugs
Muscle damage	Healing Hand	Stress, lack of potassium and magnesium, diuretics, lack of protein
Osteoporosis	Sticks and Stones	Alcohol, salty foods, coffee, carbonated drinks, smoking
Pregnancy	Earth Mother, Cool Down	Alcohol, nutritional deficiencies (especially folic acid)
Pre-menstrual tension	Berry Booster, Fine and Dandy, Bumpy Ride	Stress, junk food, alcohol, caffeine
Sinusitis	Loosen Up 1, Loosen Up 2	Smoking, alcohol, allergies, dairy foods
Stomach ulcer	Well Healed	Painkillers, poor diet, fatty food, coffee, smoking, alcohol, fizzy drinks
Thrush	Live and Kicking, Belly Berry	Coffee, antibiotics, sugar

top five fruits

Fruit	Nutrients	Benefits
Strawberries	Vitamins A, C and K, beta-carotene, folic acid, potassium	Anti-cancer, anti-viral, anti-bacterial
Apple	Vitamin C, calcium, magnesium, phosphorus, beta-carotene, pectin	Astringent, tonic, relieves constipation, reactivates beneficial gut bacteria, reduces cholesterol, helps remove toxins
Kiwifruit	Vitamin C, magnesium, phosphorus, potassium	Removes excess sodium in the body, excellent source of digestive enzymes
Orange	Vitamin C, calcium, potassium, beta-carotene, folic acid	Cleansing, internal antiseptic, stimulates peristalsis
Banana	Vitamins B6, C and K, potassium, tryptophan, beta-carotene	Promotes sleep, mild laxative, anti-fungal, natural antibiotic, helps ulcers, lowers cholesterol, helps to remove toxic metals from the body

top five vegetables

Vegetable	Nutrients	Benefits
Broccoli	Vitamins C, B3 and B5, calcium, magnesium, phosphorus, beta-carotene, folic acid	Anti-cancer, antioxidant, intestinal cleanser, excellent source of fibre, antibiotic, anti-viral, stimulates liver
Carrot	Calcium, magnesium, potassium, phosphorus, beta-carotene	Excellent detoxifier and food for the liver and digestive tract, helps kidney function, anti-viral, anti-bacterial
Cabbage	Vitamins C, E and K, calcium, magnesium, potassium, phosphorus, beta-carotene, folic acid, iodine	Eaten raw, it detoxifies the stomach and the upper colon, improves digestion, stimulates the immune system, kills bacteria and viruses. Anti-cancer, antioxidant
Beetroot	Vitamin C, calcium, magnesium, iron, phosphorus, potassium, manganese, folic acid	Good intestinal cleanser, eliminates kidney stones, blood builder, detoxifies liver and gall bladder
Tomato	Vitamin C, calcium, magnesium, phosphorus, beta-carotene, folic acid	Hydrating, antiseptic, alkaline, reduces liver inflammation, and contains lycopene which is an effective anti-cancer agent

why juice?

Vital vitamins and minerals such as antioxidants, vitamins A, B, C and E, folic acid, potassium, calcium, magnesium, zinc and amino acids are present in fresh fruits and vegetables, and are all necessary for optimum health. Because juicing removes the indigestible fibre in fruits and vegetables, the nutrients are available to the body in much larger quantities than if the piece of fruit or vegetable were eaten whole. For example, when you eat a raw carrot you are able to assimilate only about 1 per cent of the available beta-carotene because many of the nutrients are trapped in the fibre. When a carrot is juiced, thereby removing the fibre, nearly 100 per cent of the beta-carotene can be assimilated. Juicing several types of fruits and vegetables on a daily basis is therefore an easy way to ensure that your body receives its full quota of these vital vitamins and minerals.

In addition, fruits and vegetables provide another substance absolutely essential for good health — water. Most people don't consume enough water. In fact, many of the fluids we drink — coffee, tea, soft drinks, alcoholic beverages and artificially flavoured drinks — contain substances that require extra water for the body to eliminate, and tend to be dehydrating. Fruit and vegetable juices are free of these unnecessary substances.

Your health

A diet high in fruits and vegetables can prevent and help to cure a wide range of ailments. At the cutting edge of nutritional research are the plant chemicals known as phytochemicals, which hold the key

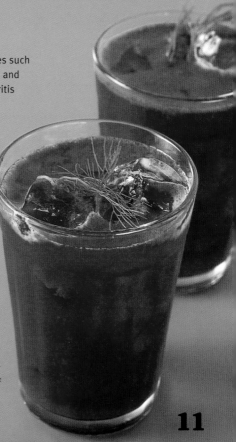

to preventing deadly diseases such as cancer and heart disease, and others such as asthma, arthritis and allergies.

Although juicing benefits your overall health, it should be used only to complement your daily eating plan. You must still eat enough from the other food groups (such as grains, dairy food and pulses) to ensure your body maintains strong bones and healthy cells. If you are following a specially prescribed diet, or are under medical supervision, you should discuss any drastic changes with your health practitioner before beginning any type of new health regime.

11

how to juice

Available in a variety of models, juicers work by separating the fruit and vegetable juice from the pulp. Choose a juicer with a reputable brand name, that has an opening big enough for larger fruits and vegetables, and make sure it is easy to take apart and clean, otherwise you may become discouraged from using it.

Types of juicer

A citrus juicer or lemon squeezer is ideal for extracting the juice from oranges, lemons, limes and grapefruit, especially if you want to add just a small amount of citrus juice to another liquid. Pure citrus juice has a high acid content, which may upset your stomach, so it is best diluted.

Centrifugal juicers are the most widely used and affordable juicers available. Fresh fruits and vegetables are fed into a rapidly spinning grater, and the pulp separated from the juice by centrifugal force. The pulp is retained in the machine while the juice runs into a separate jug. A centrifugal juicer produces less juice than the more expensive masticating juicer, which works by pulverizing fruits and vegetables, and pushing them through a wire mesh with immense force.

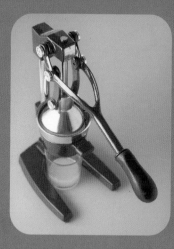

to two parts water will lessen any staining produced by the fruits and vegetables.

Preparing produce for juicing

It is best to prepare ingredients just before juicing so that fewer nutrients are lost through oxidization. Cut or tear foods into manageable pieces for juicing. If the ingredients are not organic, do not include stems, skins or roots, but if the produce is organic, you can put everything in the juicer. However, don't include the skins from pineapple, mango, papaya, citrus fruit and banana, and remove the stones from avocados, apricots, peaches, mangoes and plums. You can include melon seeds, particularly watermelon, as these are full of juice. For grape juice, choose green grapes with an amber tinge or black grapes with a darkish bloom. Leave the pith on lemons for the pectin content.

Cleaning the juicer

Clean your juicing machine thoroughly, as any residue left may harbour bacterial growth — a toothbrush or nailbrush works well for removing stubborn residual pulp. Leaving the equipment to soak in warm soapy water will loosen the residue from those hard-to-reach places. A solution made up of one part white vinegar

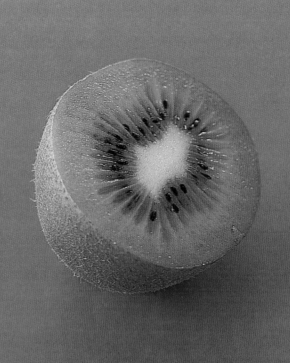

zest

THRUSH. Candida albicans is a common yeast which lives harmlessly in all of us. However, in some cases of low immunity, it can travel through the vaginal tract and cause thrush. Symptoms include mood swings and depression, recurrent vaginal yeast and chronic digestive problems. Cut out junk food, fats, sugar and highly processed foods to discourage the growth of yeast. All the ingredients in this juice have antibacterial properties. It is particularly effective if you are taking antibiotics.

live and kicking

250 g (8 oz) apple
100 g (3½ oz) frozen
   cranberries
100 g (3½ oz) live natural
   yogurt
1 tablespoon clear honey

Juice the apple and whizz in a blender with the other ingredients. Serve in a tumbler over ice cubes.
Makes 200 ml (7 fl oz)

Nutritional values

- Kcals 339
- Vitamin C 20 mg
- Calcium 40 mg

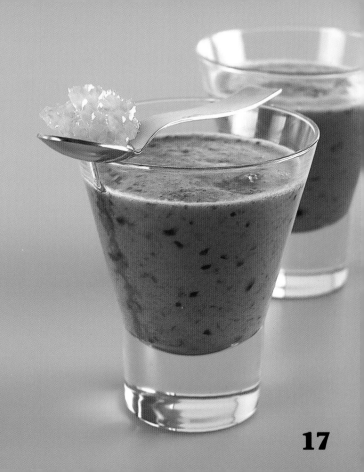

17

LOW FERTILITY. With low sperm counts and lowered fertility levels, our reproductive abilities are one of the biggest causes of concern in today's society. Male fertility may be boosted by increasing intakes of vitamin E, zinc and iron. Women should look to increase their folic acid levels, as well as zinc and vitamin E. Avocado is rich in vitamin E, while apricots are an excellent source of zinc and iron.

passion thriller

**175 g (6 oz) melon
(½ large melon)
125 g (4 oz) cucumber
125 g (4 oz) avocado
50 g (2 oz) dried apricots
1 tablespoon wheatgerm**

Juice the melon and cucumber. Whizz in a blender with the avocado, apricots, wheatgerm and a couple of ice cubes. Decorate with dried apricot slivers, if liked.

Makes 200 ml (7 fl oz)

Nutritional values

- Kcals 357
- Vitamin A 8,738 iu
- Vitamin C 110 mg
- Vitamin E 2 mcg
- Potassium 1,470 mg
- Iron 1.6 mg
- Zinc 1.29 mg

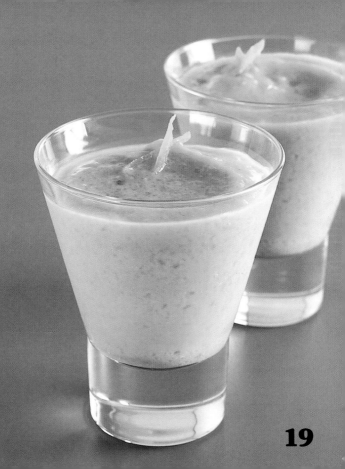

PMS. If you are one of the many women who suffer from monthly cramps, irritability and stomach upsets due to your menstrual cycle, then help is at hand! It is important to ensure that you are replacing your iron levels, as many women find that they are lethargic and tired during their period. If you also feel bloated due to water retention, or find that you gain weight just before your period, then certain fruits and vegetables may assist these symptoms. Your cycle may also affect your moods, so a calming juice may be just what you need to ensure that your cycle causes as little disruption as possible. Pineapples contain bromelain which is a great muscle relaxant, and blackberries are good sources of folic acid.

berry booster

**375 g (12 oz)
  blackberries
375 g (12 oz) pineapple
  or 1 small pineapple**

Juice the blackberries first, then the pineapple, to push through the pulp. Blend the juice with a couple of ice cubes and serve in a tall glass, decorated with a pineapple sliver, if liked.
Makes 200 ml (7 fl oz)

Nutritional values

- Kcals 353
- Vitamin A 658 iu
- Vitamin C 129.5 mg
- Iron 3.29 mg
- Potassium 1,081 mg
- Calcium 136 mg
- Folic acid 340 mcg

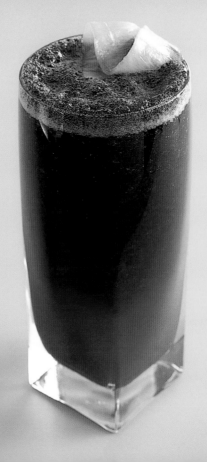

21

MENOPAUSE. The menopause occurs when the amount of the hormones oestrogen and progesterone produced by the ovaries decreases. This can be an extremely stressful time for women, as the menopause may cause irritability, hot flushes, mood swings, headaches, night sweats, vaginal dryness, loss of libido and anxiety. Beetroot is a rich source of folate which can help to protect the heart, and, together with carrots, helps to regulate hormones. Yam provides the hormone progesterone, which helps to replace the hormones lost when the menopause occurs.

cool down

175 g (6 oz) carrot
100 g (3½ oz) beetroot
175 g (6 oz) yam or
   sweet potato
125 g (4 oz) fennel

Juice all the ingredients. Mix well and serve in a glass with ice cubes. Decorate with fennel fronds, if liked.

Makes 200 ml (7 fl oz)

Nutritional values

- Kcals 296
- Vitamin A 49,430 iu
- Vitamin C 69.95 mg
- Iron 3.9 mg
- Folic acid 254 mcg
- Folate 196 mcg

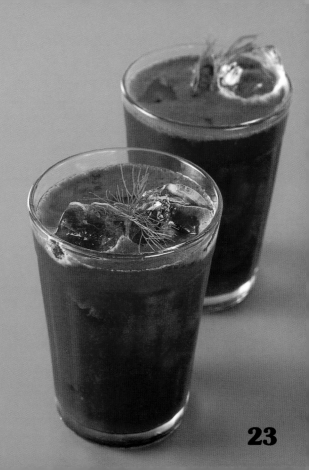

23

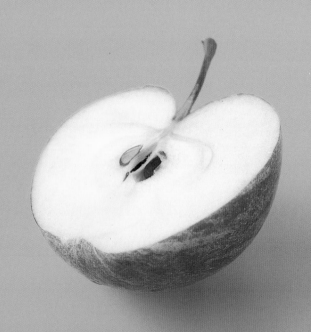

tonic

CELLULITE. The lumpy orange-peel skin that afflicts even the slimmest of women has baffled scientists and medical professionals for years. It is caused by the immobilization of fat cells, and if we eat a diet which is low in the saturated fats found in meat and dairy products this will ensure that fat cells disperse. Large amounts of water to flush out toxins, as well as fruits and vegetables with a high water content, all help to eliminate cellulite.This juice cleanses the whole system – blood, kidneys and lymph. The pectin in the apples strengthens the immune system.

bumpy ride

200 g (7 oz) apple
50 g (2 oz) beetroot
90 g (3 oz) celery

Juice together all the ingredients and serve over ice in a tumbler. Decorate with apple slices, if liked.
Makes 150 ml (¼ pint)

Nutritional values

- Kcals 179
- Vitamin A 480 iu
- Vitamin C 23 mg
- Potassium 763 mg
- Magnesium 37 mg

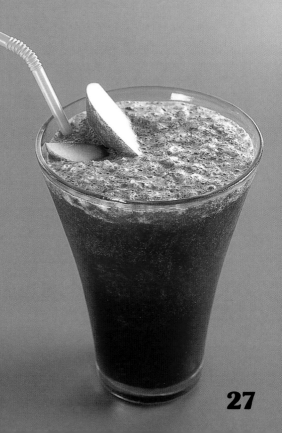

27

SINUSITIS. Sinus problems occur when the nasal and sinus passages become inflamed. Keep away from smoky places and try to avoid exhaust fumes, dust and pollen. Dairy products and wheat are also mucus-forming, so cut these out of your diet, if you can, until your condition has improved. Loosen Up 1 and Loosen Up 2 on the next page should be taken in tandem. Horseradish stimulates capillary action and dissolves mucus in the nasal passages, while the vitamin C in lemon juice may help to lower a high temperature.

loosen up 1

1½ teaspoons pulverized horseradish
½ lemon

Pulverize the horseradish by juicing a small amount and mixing the juice and the pulp. Put it into a shot glass and stir in the lemon juice. Take twice a day.
Makes 50 ml (2 fl oz)

Nutritional values

- Kcals 25
- Vitamin C 55 mg
- Selenium 0.4 mcg
- Zinc 0.18 mg

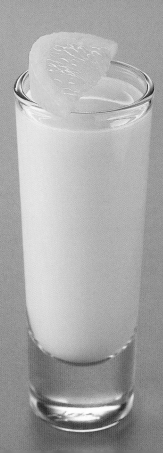

29

SINUSITIS. This juice should be taken one hour after Loosen Up 1 on page 30. The radish juice is too strong to be taken alone, but combined with carrot it has the effect of soothing the membranes and cleansing the body of the mucus dissolved by the horseradish in Loosen Up 1.

loosen up 2

175 g (6 oz) carrot
100 g (3½ oz) radishes,
with tops and leaves
2.5 cm (1 inch) cube
fresh root ginger,
roughly chopped
(optional)

Juice the carrot, radishes and ginger, if using. Add some ice cubes. Drink one hour after Loosen Up 1.
Makes 200 ml (7 fl oz)

Nutritional values

- Kcals 115
- Vitamin A 49,233 iu
- Vitamin C 40 mg
- Selenium 2.82 mcg
- Zinc 0.8 mg

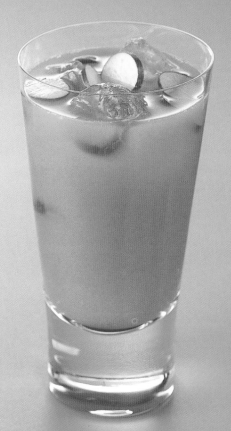

31

BLOATING OR WATER RETENTION. This can be uncomfortable and painful. The problem can be caused by food allergies, hormonal imbalances, a lack of essential fatty acids in the diet, and also, ironically, by not drinking enough water. All the ingredients in this juice contain high levels of zinc and potassium. This recipe is also great if you have just eaten a salty meal. Zinc is essential to decrease water retention.

fine and dandy

125 g (4 oz) asparagus spears
10 dandelion leaves
125 g (4 oz) melon
175 g (6 oz) cucumber
200 g (7 oz) pear

Trim the woody bits off the asparagus spears. Roll the dandelion leaves into a ball and juice them (if you have picked wild leaves, wash them first) with the asparagus. Peel and juice the melon. Juice the cucumber and pear with their skins. Whizz everything in a blender and serve in a tall glass with ice cubes.

Makes 200 ml (7 fl oz)

Nutritional values

- Kcals 215
- Vitamin A 5,018 iu
- Vitamin C 87 mg
- Potassium 1,235 mg
- Zinc 1.36 mg

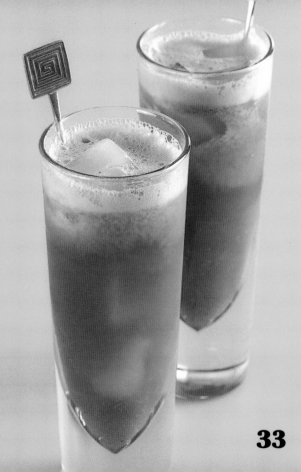

33

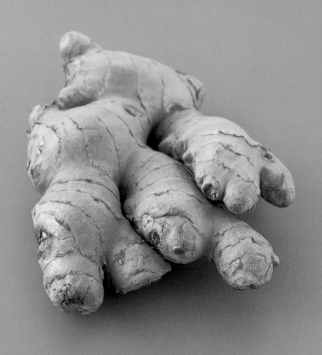

wellbeing

HEART DISEASE. This is one of the most preventable diseases in today's society. An increased intake of fried and fatty foods, a high salt intake, stress, smoking and lack of exercise are all contributory factors. Boosting your intake of vitamin C and vitamin E and taking regular exercise can add as many as ten years to your life. The onion and garlic thin the blood and help to lower cholesterol. Watercress oxygenates the blood and beetroot builds up the red blood cells.

heart beet

125 g (4 oz) beetroot
125 g (4 oz) watercress
125 g (4 oz) red onion
250 g (8 oz) carrot
1 garlic clove

Juice the ingredients and serve in a tall glass. Decorate with beet leaves and watercress, if liked.

Makes 200 ml (7 fl oz)

Nutritional values

- Kcals 167
- Vitamin A 41,166 iu
- Vitamin C 85 mg
- Magnesium 85 mg
- Niacin 2 mg
- Vitamin B6 0.56 mg
- Vitamin E 2.36 mg

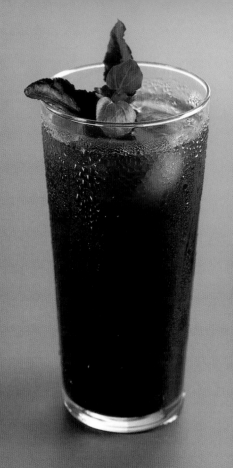

37

REDUCING CHOLESTEROL. High cholesterol levels are caused by eating a diet containing too much saturated fat, which leads to a build-up along the inside walls of the arteries. Grapefruit is particularly recommended for its rich source of vitamin C and bioflavonoids, which protect the health of the arteries. Blueberries are also extremely potent antioxidants and, along with apples, can help prevent hardening of the arteries and reduce cholesterol levels.

purple passion

250 g (8 oz) blueberries
125 g (4 oz) grapefruit
250 g (8 oz) apple
2.5 cm (1 inch) cube
  fresh root ginger,
  roughly chopped

Juice all the ingredients and serve in a tall glass with ice cubes. Decorate with thin slices of ginger, if liked.

Makes 200 ml (7 fl oz)

Nutritional values

- Kcals 380
- Vitamin A 695 iu
- Vitamin C 134 mg
- Magnesium 59 mg
- Niacin 1.91 mg
- Vitamin B6 0.39 mg
- Vitamin E 3.12 mg

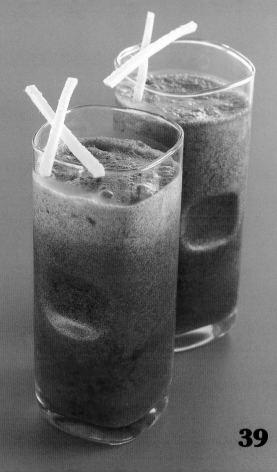

ANAEMIA. If you lack iron in your diet (possibly due to a vegetarian diet, or a heavy menstrual cycle) then you may have anaemia, which can leave you feeling lethargic, depressed, or prone to flu and colds. Folic acid builds up red blood cells, chlorophyll helps to combat fatigue, and spirulina provides a valuable boost of vitamin B12.

iron maiden

250 g (8 oz) spinach
25 g (1 oz) parsley
250 g (8 oz) carrot
1 teaspoon spirulina

Juice the spinach, parsley and carrot and stir in the spirulina. Serve in a tumbler, decorated with carrot slivers, if liked.
Makes 200 ml (7 fl oz)

Nutritional values

- Kcals 229
- Vitamin C 450 mg
- Folic acid 235 mg
- Chlorophyll 100 mg
- Vitamin B12 20 mcg

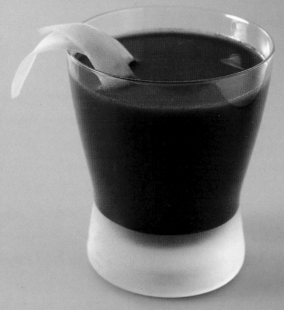

41

MOTION SICKNESS. If even the thought of travelling by boat or plane, or by any form of transport which has a constant rocking motion, makes you feel queasy then a fresh ginger juice may provide the solution. (One teaspoon of dried ginger in apple juice works well, if you are on the move.) Said to be more effective than anything else you can buy over the counter, ginger is ideal for quelling nausea. Drink just before travelling.

quantum leap

250 g (8 oz) apple
2.5 cm (1 inch) cube
   fresh root ginger,
   roughly chopped

Juice the apple and ginger and serve in a glass over ice. Decorate with apple slices, if liked. This drink can be diluted with sparkling mineral water to taste.
Makes 100 ml (3½ fl oz)

Nutritional values

- Kcals 160
- Vitamin C 16 mg

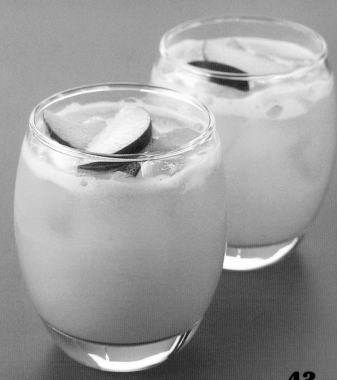

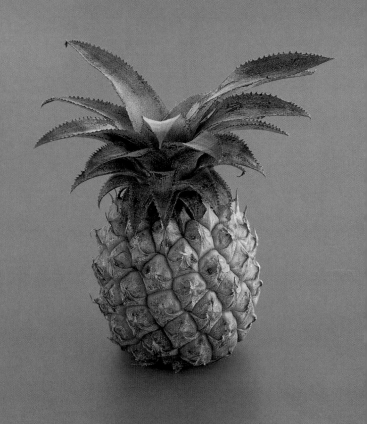

vitality

STOMACH ULCERS. These are caused by excess acid and the digestive enzyme pepsin and are aggravated by stress, smoking and acidic food and drinks. They can be controlled by keeping your intake as alkaline as possible, but if you have severe abdominal pain you must always consult a doctor. Both carrot and cabbage juices are renowned for having a healing effect on stomach ulcers.

well healed

250 g (8 oz) carrot
**250 g (8 oz) green
   cabbage**

Juice the vegetables and serve in a tumbler over ice.
Makes 200 ml (7 fl oz)

Nutritional values

- Kcals 180
- Vitamin A 70,654 iu
- Vitamin C 105 mg
- Selenium 5 mcg
- Zinc 0.95 mg

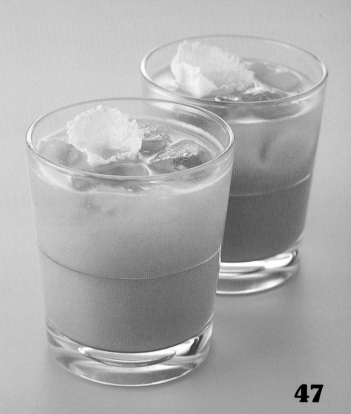

47

CONSTIPATION. A sluggish digestive system, caused by poor diet and lack of digestive enzymes, can cause constipation, an uncomfortable affliction which may lead to blockage and distension of the bowel. A combination of fruit and vegetables high in fibre and cleansing properties will help to exercise and stimulate the abdomen and improve digestion. This juice really could be called a lethal weapon – a dose of three potent laxatives that will get you back on line.

way to go

250 g (8 oz) pear
25 g (1 oz) pitted prunes
125 g (4 oz) spinach

Juice all the ingredients and serve in a glass over ice cubes. Decorate with pear slices, if liked.
Makes 200 ml (7 fl oz)

Nutritional values

- Kcals 302
- Vitamin A 8,946 iu
- Vitamin C 80 mg
- Potassium 1,311 mg

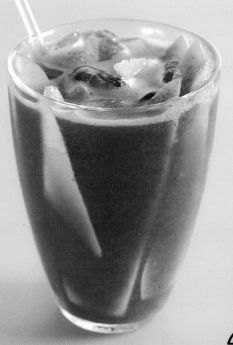

49

DIARRHOEA. Whether you're suffering from food poisoning, stress, travel sickness or jet-lag, diarrhoea will dehydrate your system. This means you must ensure that your body gets plenty of liquids to replace the nutrients lost. Blueberries contain anthocyanosides, which are lethal to the bacteria that can cause diarrhoea.

belly berry

250 g (8 oz) apple
125 g (4 oz) blueberries,
  fresh or frozen

Juice the apple, then whizz in a blender with the blueberries. Serve in a tumbler.
Makes 150 ml (¼ pint)

Nutritional values

- Kcals 210
- Vitamin A 8.946 iu
- Vitamin C 20 mg
- Magnesium 18.5 mg

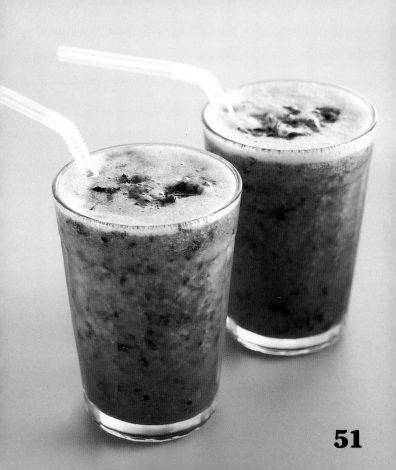

ARTHRITIS. The most common form of arthritis, whereby the smooth layer of cartilage that covers and cushions the ends of the bones gradually breaks down, mainly affects elderly people. The swollen and inflamed joints that result are an extremely painful condition. There are many foods that can ease the discomfort of this complaint including cabbage, citrus fruits, berries and fruits high in vitamin C. The salicylic acid in grapefruit works to break down uric acid deposits and the carrot and spinach help to rebuild and regenerate cartilage and joints.

twister

125 g (4 oz) pink grapefruit
125 g (4 oz) carrot
125 g (4 oz) spinach

Peel the grapefruit, keeping as much of the pith as possible. Juice all the ingredients and serve in a tumbler. Decorate with slices of grapefruit, if liked.
Makes 200 ml (7 fl oz)

Nutritional values

- Kcals 185
- Vitamin A 43,864 iu
- Vitamin C 167 mg
- Cysteine 43 mg

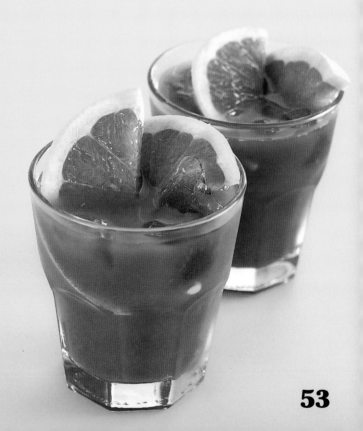

53

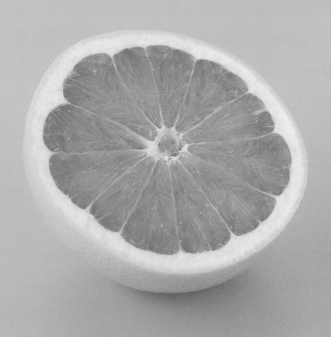

fitness

OSTEOPOROSIS. This is a debilitating disease, and, although it primarily affects women who have gone through the menopause, it is imperative that even women in their twenties supplement their eating plan with bone-strengthening foods. Turnip-top leaves contain more calcium than milk. Broccoli is also ideal, as it also contains calcium and folic acid. Dandelion leaves are excellent sources of magnesium, which helps the body utilize the calcium for healthy bones and teeth.

sticks and stones

125 g (4 oz) turnip, including the tops
125 g (4 oz) carrot
125 g (4 oz) broccoli
handful of dandelion leaves
175 g (6 oz) apple

Scrub the turnip and carrot. Juice all the ingredients and whizz in a blender with a couple of ice cubes. Serve in a tall glass decorated with dandelion leaves, if liked.
Makes 200 ml (7 fl oz)

Nutritional values

- Kcals 196
- Vitamin A 50,391 iu
- Vitamin C 223 mg
- Magnesium 108 mg
- Calcium 398 mg
- Folic acid 210 mcg

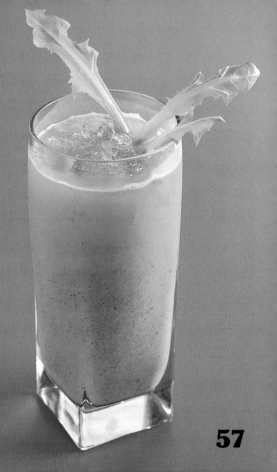

57

EYESIGHT. Remember when your mother nagged you to eat your carrots, so that you could see in the dark? Well, she was right, as carrots contain high levels of beta-carotene and vitamin E, which are necessary for maintaining healthy eyes. Endive is helpful in preventing cataracts. This combination of vegetables provides a high vitamin A content that nourishes the optic nerve.

vision impeccable

175 g (6 oz) carrot
125 g (4 oz) endive
125 g (4 oz) celery

Juice the carrot, endive and celery. Whizz in a blender with a couple of ice cubes and serve decorated with lemon slices and some chopped parsley, if liked.
Makes 200 ml (7 fl oz)

Nutritional values

- Kcals 128
- Vitamin A 53,687 iu
- Vitamin C 33 mg
- Potassium 1,499 mg

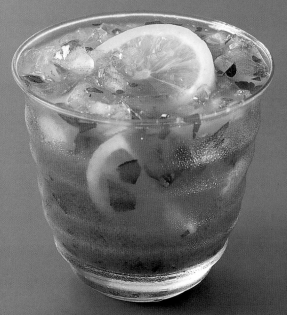

59

PREGNANCY CARE. Eating (or juicing) for two may seem overwhelming when you are first pregnant, but you do not need to double your intake of nutrients and vitamins although it is recommended that you increase several of them. Nutritionists advise that, for most women, an additional 200 calories per day is all that's required therefore juicing is a great way to increase your intake of nutrients whilst controlling your calorie count. More importantly, though, ensure that you eat (or juice) foods high in folic acid, to reduce the possibility of spina bifida. This juice is rich in folic acid and vitamin A, which are essential for foetal development and guard against pre-eclampsia.

earth mother

125 g (4 oz) carrot
125 g (4 oz) lettuce
125 g (4 oz) parsnip
125 g (4 oz) cantaloupe melon

Juice the carrot, lettuce and parsnip with the flesh of the melon. Serve in a tall glass with wedges of melon, if liked.
Makes 200 ml (7 fl oz)

Nutritional values

- Kcals 204
- Vitamin A 42,136 iu
- Vitamin C 115 mg
- Folic acid 93.75 mcg
- Fat 2.1 g

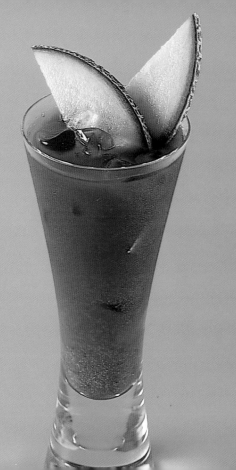

61

MUSCLE DAMAGE. Athletes often suffer muscle damage during training and, even with precautions, often seem to attract bangs, knocks and other injuries. Ensuring that there is enough vitamin C in your diet helps protect against muscle damage, and leads to a reduction in muscle soreness and improved general healing. Vitamin C may also help to increase oxygen uptake and aerobic energy production. Weight for weight, kiwifruits contain more vitamin C than oranges.

healing hand

2 ripe pears
3 kiwifruits
½ lime

Wash the pears, peel the kiwifruits and scrub the lime. Slice the fruit into even-sized pieces then juice. Pour into a glass, add a couple of ice cubes and decorate with slices of kiwifruit, if liked.
Makes 300 ml (½ pint)

Nutritional values

- Kcals 210
- Protein 3 g
- Vitamin C 130 mg
- Calcium 80 mg
- Iron 1.3 mg

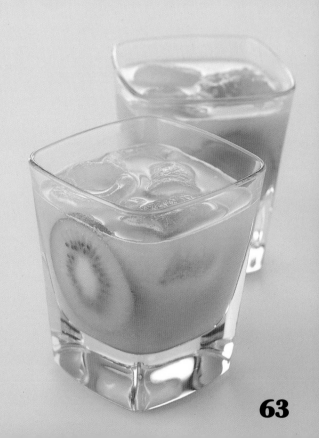

63

index

acknowledgements

The publisher would like to thank The Juicer Company
for the loan of The Champion juicer and the Orange X
citrus juicer (featured on pages 12 and 13).

The Juicer Company
28 Shambles
York
YO1 7LX
Tel: (01904) 541541
www.thejuicercompany.co.uk

Executive Editor Nicola Hill
Editor Rachel Lawrence
Executive Art Editor Geoff Fennell
Designer Sue Michniewicz
Senior Production Controller Jo Sim
Photographer Stephen Conroy
Home Economist David Morgan
Stylist Angela Swaffield
All photographs © Octopus
Publishing Group Ltd